Atkins Diet

Dr. Atkins New Diet Revolution
6 Week Low Carb Diet Plan for You

Table of Content

CHAPTER 1. Introduction 1
CHAPTER 2. Atkins Diet and Weight Loss 5
CHAPTER 3. Phases of Atkins Diet 7
CHAPTER 4. Which Foods Should be Eaten and Which Should be Restricted 9
CHAPTER 5. Atkins Six Weeks Diet Plan 12
CHAPTER 6. Safety and Effectiveness of Atkins Diet 40
CHAPTER 7. Recipes for Atkins Diet 43
CHAPTER 8. Frequently Asked Questions 45
CHAPTER 9. Conclusion 46

CHAPTER 1. Introduction

Atkins diet gets its name from Dr. Robert Coleman Atkins (October 17, 1930—April 17, 2003), who was a cardiologist and an American physician. He was 224 pounds (100kg) when he decided to follow a diet pattern based on the research of Dr. Alfred W. Pennington and found success in achieving his target weight.

According to this diet pattern, all food sources of starch and sugars need to be restricted. He achieved success for himself after following this diet and then, became a strong and vocal advocate of it for others. He started promoting it among his overweight patients, achieved success in this with sixty-five of his patients, and helped them reduce weight through this diet regimen.

Later on, he promoted it through media and this diet started gaining recognition and popularity. Atkins diet meal plans and books were published. Atkins commercial products became popular, widely available, and part of promotion for alternative therapies. Later on, Dr. Atkins revised his weight loss plan and dietary approach to add more room for flexibility and variety.

Atkins diet is all about a low carbohydrate, moderate fat, and high protein diet. The basic idea behind this kind of diet is to promote catabolism of adipose tissues, or in other words, the break down and utilization of fat deposits and fat stores of the body, while encouraging anabolism of muscle tissues or build-up of more muscle mass.

The process of ketosis is encouraged so that instead of relying on carbohydrates and glucose as primary sources of energy, the body gets adapted to utilize fats for energy. In this, ketone bodies are used to furnish energy instead of glucose. Our brain prefers the energy of glucose over any other source of energy, but in the absence of glucose, it learn to adapt itself and utilizes the energy of ketones furnished through metabolism of fats.

A diet high in protein and moderate in fat helps in providing satiety for a longer period of time than a diet with high carbohydrates; consequently, less amount of food is being consumed. Glucose energy supports fat anabolism or build-up of fat stores inside the body. In the absence of carbohydrates, our body learns to adapt and utilize other available sources of energy in normal conditions, as well as in fasting, starvation, and dietary regimen changes.

Atkins diet or Atkins Nutrition Approach limits the consumption of carbohydrates and switches the body's metabolism towards lipolysis. Dr. Atkins' theory that a low carbohydrate diet produces a kind of metabolic advantage was considered controversial and later on, this aspect was altered and to some extent removed, as many health practitioners disagreed and did not want to be a part of this theory, as they considered lower calories were being consumed due to boredom, simplicity and monotony of the diet which inhibited the appetite and overall food intake.

Atkins diet should be planned so that no more than 20% of the calories come from saturated fats. This diet is divided into four different phases and the initial phase, called the induction phase, resembles that of a ketogenic diet.

There have been few conclusive studies suggesting that Atkins diet may be helpful in the prevention of cardiovascular diseases and lowering LDL (bad type) cholesterol while increasing HDL (good type cholesterol). There also have been some studies suggesting this diet may contribute towards osteoporosis and kidney diseases.

The four phases of this diet include the induction phase, ongoing weight loss phase, pre-maintenance phase, and lifetime maintenance phase.

When you plan to opt for Atkins diet, keep focused and set goals. Understand the diet and how it works. Committing may mean facing resistance and having the willpower to achieve your desired weight goal. Persistence, adaptability in meal planning, proper approach, and right guidance is needed. Motivation is the key to success and motivation should be your driving force. If possible, plan it in a group so that you are able to discuss it with people going through the same thing. Get mentally prepared and familiarize yourself with the allowed and restricted list of food items.

Visualize your planning and learn the art of developing creativity in meal planning and recipe development. Learn to stay hydrated at all times. Restricting fat in this diet is not recommended and you may feel free to include fried food items, as well as good sources of fats in your daily meal plan. Snacking is encouraged, therefore, think of all the ways to have healthy snacks that adhere to the boundaries of Atkins diet. Keep yourself satisfied through small frequent meals, so that you do not feel hungry and go back to your previous high carbohydrate diet.

Atkins is all about limiting your total carbohydrates, rather than omitting them. It also helps in encouraging the use of more fibrous and nutritious sources of vegetables, rather than limiting yourself to the starchy ones. Many published research studies confirm Atkins diet's safety, as well as efficacy. Atkins is not only easy, but it is also a great-tasting and fulfilling way of weight loss.

Starting with phase 1 is ideal for weight loss, but you can also start with phase 2, or even from phase 3, as well. If you are starting with phase 1, you must start with limiting your intake of carbohydrates to 20 grams/day. Divide these 20 grams among all the meals that you will be consuming. You may achieve maximum weight loss this way. If you are planning to skip phase 1 and start with phase 2, than you should limit your carbohydrate intake to 25 to 30 grams/day. In this way, it will take longer for you to lose weight. If you have very little weight to lose or want to lose weight slowly, then you may even opt to start from phase 3. In this, you will have to consume 45 grams of total carbohydrates/day.

Whatever way you may choose, it is advisable to spread out all your meals in five small meals, rather than three large ones. Do not overeat, and eat just enough to keep your body contented and satisfied. Follow the recommended guidelines for dietary planning. Irregular diet pattern may lessen your likelihood of losing weight. Consistency is needed once you plan to go ahead with it for overall good results. Your blood sugar will start stabilizing from day five and your cravings for carbohydrate rich sources of foods may reduce. At least 12 to 15 grams of your total carbohydrates in the induction phase should come from the foundation vegetables.

Atkins diet emphasizes counting your net carbohydrate intake. Carbohydrates are of two types: digestible or indigestible. It can also be defined as complex carbohydrates and simple sugars. Fiber is a carbohydrate comprised of two types: soluble and insoluble. Both types of fibers are not digested and therefore, get excreted.

All vegetables that are allowed on an Atkins diet do contain fiber, as well as digestible carbohydrates, in the form of complex carbohydrates, such as starch and simple sugars. When we say net carbohydrates, we mean subtracting the fiber part from any given carbohydrates. Therefore 20 grams carbohydrates mean only the starch and sugar that any given vegetable may contain. If a cup of any given vegetable contains 3.5 grams of total carbohydrates and 2 grams fiber that means we are getting 1.5 gram of net carbohydrates that will supply us with glucose energy.

CHAPTER 2. Atkins Diet and Weight Loss

Atkins diet is one of the most popular weight reducing diets. The weight loss program starts with the induction phase which lasts for two weeks, and you can lose up to 15 pounds in this phase. After this initial phase, you have to pass through a systematic procedure of finding your personal carbohydrate balance that you can consume while you continue to lose weight.

You need to keep your appetite under control and stay energized and alert. All high carbohydrate food sources are at first limited and gradually increased in a controlled manner. Meat, fish, poultry, cheese, fats and oils, and low carbohydrate, low starch vegetables are the main content of this diet pattern.

Having seen peak popularity during the year 2002, it still is considered one of the most popularly selected pattern of weight loss. Many Atkins low carbohydrates products are still available for use and learning the basics may help in diet and menu planning to suit individual needs.

In this, a high protein diet is being encouraged to furnish the energy requirements of the body. Steaks, roasts, BBQ, grilled, fried foods are the main sources of calories and any method of cooking can be applied due to the liberal fat content of this diet. Incorporating allowed vegetables in an interesting manner can be challenging.

Vegetables are a good source of minerals, vitamins and fiber. Vegetables, e.g. leafy greens, cucumbers, beans, broccoli, tomatoes, cauliflower, cabbage, eggplant, zucchini, onions, peppers, olives, and peas are all rich in minerals, vitamins, and fiber and are low carbohydrates vegetables Therefore, these need to be incorporated in a variety of ways, especially fresh salads.

You may have to restrict your carbohydrates to 20 grams/day initially and you may find it difficult to stick to this kind of diet at times. Carbohydrates are restricted to encourage lipolysis or break down of fat. You start burning your fat stores when you control your carbohydrates intake. Another reason for weight loss is due to the feeling of satisfaction for a longer period of time and not frequently feeling hungry.

Another reason behind the popularity of this diet is that you lose weight without having to exercise. It also encourages the intake of carbohydrates progressively. It is easy to stick with, as many interesting food items are being promoted and encouraged. Actual weight loss occurring may vary for each and every individual.

CHAPTER 3. Phases of Atkins Diet

Four phases of Atkins diet include the following:

Induction phase is the most restrictive of all Atkins diet phases. It lasts for two weeks. It is intended to allow the body to enter in the state of ketosis. Total carbohydrates are restricted to less than 20 grams net per day from the vegetables allowed list. This phase encourages the use of protein and fat rich sources of foods. Eight glasses of water is recommended. Moderate intake of caffeine is also allowed.

Have three or more small meals. Try not to reduce or increase your total carbohydrates to less than 18 grams or more than 22 grams on a daily basis. Eat enough protein to encourage fat loss and eventually, weight loss and muscle build up. Initially, you may lose a great amount of body water which may lead to lightheadedness and other related symptoms. Most of these symptoms will start disappearing as you progress towards burning fat primarily.

To replace water loss and to avoid dehydration, drink enough water and liquids, which may include clear broth, soups and unsweetened beverages. These liquids will help you in maintaining the electrolyte balance of the body. Try to avoid commercially prepared food items and eating out. If you absolutely must eat out, be certain of the ingredients used. Be watchful of the hidden sources of carbohydrates. You may use sugar substitutes, but limit intake to 1 to 3 packets per day.

You may use commercial products especially designed for Atkins and the majority of them can be used during the induction phase. If you plan to continue phase 1 for more than two weeks, then you may add on the nuts and seeds, in addition to your present meal plan. To conclude, in order to kickstart phase 1, include the foundation vegetables, proteins, fats, and cheeses.

Ongoing weight loss (OWL) phase consists of incremental increases in carbohydrate intake. Usually 5 grams of carbohydrate intake is increased on a weekly basis. Sources of carbohydrates are increased gradually, keeping in mind not to trigger carbohydrate cravings. This phase lasts until weight is within 4.5 kg (10 pounds) of the target weight.

The ladder of nine rungs of carbohydrate sources of foods are increased in a systematic manner. As we proceed from phase 1 to phase 2, we may start to increase our carbohydrate intake by adding more carbohydrate food sources, beginning with nuts and seeds and proceeding with other sources accordingly, which may include berries, cherries and melon, whole milk, Greek cheese, yogurt, ricotta cheese, cottage cheese, legumes and tomato juice. After the induction period is over start adding more vegetables, nuts, seeds, cheeses, coconut milk, soy milk, almond milk.

Pre-maintenance phase allows increasing carbohydrates by 10 grams each week progressively and the key goal in this is to find the "Critical Carbohydrate Level for Maintenance". Some of the forbidden carbohydrates will start to reappear in the meals gradually on a weekly basis. During the third phase of fine tuning, you may become more liberal in your total carbohydrate intake progressively and gradually. Start by adding additional fruits, then progress to add starchy vegetables, and finally, begin adding the whole grain cereals.

Lifetime maintenance phase is mainly intended to support and carry the acquired habits during previous phases. If you start to follow the original habits, then you will have to go back again to your previous phase.

CHAPTER 4. Which Foods Should be Eaten and Which Should be Restricted

Foods which are considered to be **allowed** on Atkins diet includes all types of **fish** e. g. cod, trout, halibut, tuna, sole, flounder, salmon, herring, sardines, etc.

All **shellfish** are also allowed, which may include lobster, shrimp, mussels, squid, oysters, crab, clams, and prawns.

All types of **meat** may also be included, such as veal, beef, mutton, chicken, lamb, quail, duck and turkey.

Eggs in all styles and forms may also be a part of this diet. Fried, soft-boiled, hard-boiled, omelets, poached, scrambled or any other sort of eggs are all fine.

All types of **cheese** may be included, like Swiss, feta, mozzarella, parmesan, cream cheese, gouda, cheddar, blue cheeses, etc.

Many low carbohydrate **vegetables** are allowed in limited amounts, including bokchoy, alfalfa sprouts, arugula, celery, chicory green, chives, jicama, fennel, escarole, endive, daikon, cucumber, green leaf lettuce, radishes, radicchio, peppers, parsley, mushrooms, and iceberg lettuce.

Theapproved **vegetable** list may also include vegetables which are slightly higher in carbohydrates, such as cabbage, Brussels sprouts, broccoflower, broccoli, bamboo shoots, avocados, artichoke hearts, asparagus, cauliflower, Swiss chard, collard greens, eggplant, green string beans, okra, leeks, kohlrabi, kale, hearts of palm, olives, onion, pumpkin, rhubarb, sauerkraut, snow peas, snap peas, spaghetti squash, spinach, tomatoes, turnips, water chestnuts, and zucchini.

All **herbs and spices** may be included as required, only make sure that they are in their original form without any additives. Spices and herbs allowed include tarragon, sage, rosemary, pepper, oregano, basil, cayenne pepper, cilantro, dill, garlic, and ginger.

No added sugar and low carbohydrate **salad dressings** are also allowed, like lime juice, lemon juice, oil and vinegar, Italian, Caesar, blue cheese, etc.

Fats and oils in the allowed list include butter, olive oil, mayonnaise, sesame seeds oil, walnut oil, almond oil, coconut oil, grape-seed oil, sunflower oil, safflower oil and all other vegetable oils.

Splenda may be used sparingly and 1 packet contains 1 gram of carbohydrates.

Beverages that are on the allowed list include decaffeinated tea and coffee, clear broth, cream, both heavy and light, diet soda, herbal teas, unsweetened and unflavored soy milk and almond milk. Make sure to include eight glasses of water or substitutes of water in the form of other fluids e.g. broth, tea, etc.

Foods restricted on Atkins diet include whole grain cereals and all products containing these, like cakes, biscuits, buns, bread, pastries, pitas, fruits, fruit juices, all fruit products, milk, potatoes, sweet potatoes, beets, corn, legumes, alcoholic beverages, nuts and seeds.

Oysters and mussels needed to be limited to 4 ounces per day as comparatively these are higher in carbohydrate content. Processed meat may contain sugar, therefore try to avoid these. Add eggs to your breakfast meal on a daily basis, as these are considered a staple on Atkins diet. Be creative with all the recipes, especially breakfast egg recipes and add vegetables, like onions, peppers or mushrooms. Make it more fulfilling by adding your choice of cheese.

Use herbs and spices liberally to add flavor and aroma whenever and wherever needed. Cheeses do contain carbohydrates, around 1 gram per ounce, therefore you may include 3 to 4 ounces of it initially on a daily basis. A one inch cube of cheese is around one ounce. Initially, you may use three to four cups of mixed vegetables. One cup of raw vegetables is equal to around half cup of cooked vegetables. Or you may use 4 cups of raw salads and 2 cups of cooked vegetables from your foundation vegetables. A one inch cube of boneless meat is around one ounce in weight. Each individuals' food needs may differ, according to individual height, weight and activity factor.

CHAPTER 5. Atkins Six Weeks Diet Plan

PHASE 1, FIRST WEEK AND SECOND WEEK DIET PLAN

(12 ounces to 18 ounces meat source of protein, 1 to 2 eggs, 20 grams net carbohydrates which means around 120–200 grams of salads and 100–150 grams of cooked vegetables or 3 to 4 cups of salads and 2 cups of cooked vegetables per day, oils and fats as required or needed, 2 to 3 ounces of cheese, 1 cup of coconut water)

DAY 1

BREAKFAST

Cheese omelet with olives

Roasted mixed vegetables with coconut butter

Decaffeinated green tea with Splenda

MID MORNING SNACK

Cucumber slices

LUNCH

Chicken and vegetables clear soup

Fried fish with lemon sauce

Fresh sliced salad

AFTERNOON SNACK

Coconut water

DINNER

Onion cream soup

Beef Kebabs

Lettuce and cucumber diced salad

DAY 2

BREAKFAST

Scrambled eggs with mixed vegetables

Earl grey tea

MID MORNING SNACK
Cucumber slices

LUNCH
Mushrooms and cream cheese soup

Roast chicken with grilled peppers

Cole slaw

AFTERNOON SNACK
Coconut water

DINNER
Chicken and vegetables cream soup

Fried mutton chops with stir fried bean sprouts

Fresh green salad

DAY 3

BREAKFAST
Baked egg with sausage and vegetables

Lemon tea

MID MORNING SNACK
Cucumber slices

LUNCH
Beef and vegetables soup

Chicken steak with cream cheese

Mixed vegetables salad

AFTERNOON SNACK
Coconut water

DINNER
Bean, chicken and cream soup

Baked fish with beans and stirfried bean sprouts

Cucumber and lettuce salad

DAY 4
BREAKFAST
Cheese omelet

Stirfried Vegetables

Tea

MID MORNING SNACK
Cucumber slices

LUNCH
Egg, tomato, and pepper soup

Mutton and mixed vegetables stew

Cherry tomatoes and olives

DINNER
Chicken BBQ

Mixed vegetables cutlet

Fresh iceberg lettuce diced with dressing

DAY 5
BREAKFAST
Cheese, sausage and vegetables omelet

Tea

MID MORNING SNACK
Cucumber slices

LUNCH
Mutton and vegetables clear soup

Chicken and vegetables stirfried with peanut butter

Mixed vegetables, dressed salad

AFTERNOON SNACK
Coconut water

DINNER
Chicken clear soup

Baked fish

Vegetables cutlet

DAY 7
BREAKFAST
Scrambled eggs with vegetables

Tea

MID MORNING SNACK
Cucumber slices

LUNCH
Egg, tomato and onion soup

Grilled chicken with peanut butter

Baked mixed vegetables

AFTERNOON SNACK
Coconut water

DINNER
Chicken vegetables cream soup

Fried fish with coconut butter

Fresh mixed diced salad with lemon dressing

DAY 8
BREAKFAST
Cheese omelet

Roasted vegetables

Tea

MID MORNING SNACK
Cucumber slices

LUNCH
Beef clear soup

Grilled chicken with cream cheese

Sliced fresh salad

AFTERNOON SNACK
Coconut water

DINNER
Mixed vegetables and chicken soup

Baked fish with coconut cream

Tomato and cucumber salad

DAY 9

BREAKFAST
Fried egg

Vegetables cutlet

Tea

MID MORNING SNACK
Cucumber slices

LUNCH
Bean and chicken soup

Beef steak with avocado, lemon and cream sauce

Diced mixed salad with olive oil dressing

AFTERNOON SNACK
Coconut water

DINNER
Cream of beef and vegetables soup

Fried chicken with mayo garlic sauce

Roast mixed vegetables with sesame seed oil

DAY 10

BREAKFAST
Baked egg with cheese and vegetables

Tea

MID MORING SNACK
Cucumber slices

LUNCH
Chicken, bell pepper and cream cheese soup

Baked mutton chops with mayo garlic sauce

Grilled mixed vegetables with olive oil

AFTERNOON SNACK
Coconut water

DINNER
Beef and vegetables cream soup

Baked chicken with baked vegetables

Fresh sliced salad with mayo dressing

DAY 11

BREAKFAST
Scrambled eggs with cheese and vegetables

Tea

MID MORNING SNACK
Cucumber slices

LUNCH
Mixed vegetables and chicken cream soup

Grilled chicken with grilled vegetables

Mixed salad with sesame seed oil and lemon dressing

AFTERNOON SNACK
Coconut water

DINNER
Beef and vegetables cream soup

Roast beef with roast vegetables

Fresh green salad with coconut oil and vinegar dressing

DAY 12
BREAKFAST
Fried egg with fried tofu

Grilled mixed vegetables

Tea

MID MORNING SNACK
Cucumber slices

LUNCH
Mushroom and onion cream soup

Fried fish with cream cheese and mayo garlic sauce

Mixed diced salad with mustard sauce

AFTERNOON SNACK
Coconut water

DINNER
Chicken and avocado cream soup

Baked chicken with sour stirfried vegetables

Mixed vegetables bowl with lemon and mint dressing

DAY 13
BREAKFAST
Fried sausages, egg and stirfried vegetables and cream cheese

Tea

MID MORNING SNACK
Cucumber slices

LUNCH
Clear chicken and vegetables soup

Stirfried chicken with sautéed broccoli

Diced cucumber with mayo garlic dressing

AFTERNOON SNACK
Coconut water

DINNER
Beef and vegetables cream soup

Beef and vegetables with cream cheese and spaghetti squash

Sliced and dressed mixed salad

DAY 14

BREAKFAST
Baked egg with tofu, cheese and vegetables

Tea

MID MORNING SNACK
Cucumber slices

LUNCH
Cream of broccoli and chicken soup

Fried prawns with grilled spicy vegetables

Sliced dressed avocado

AFTERNOON SNACK
Coconut water

DINNER
Broccoli and tomato cream soup

Baked salmon with tomato cream sauce

Avocado slices with olive oil and lemon dressing

Phase 2, THIRD WEEK DIET PLAN

In the second phase of Atkins diet, you may start adding 5 grams of net carbohydrates on a weekly basis. You may have net 25 grams of carbohydrates in the third week or first week of second phase. Begin by adding one ounce or a hand full of nuts (peanuts, walnuts, almonds, pecans, pistachios, macadamias, Brazil nuts) or one ounce of seeds (sunflower seeds or pumpkin seeds). Also start adding ¼ to ½ a cup of raspberries or strawberries in addition to all the food you are allowed in phase 1.

Day 15

BREAKFAST

Hard-boiled egg with cream cheese

Fried sausages with scrambled eggs and stirfried vegetables

Tea

MID MORNING SNACK
Mixed nuts

LUNCH

Clear chicken and vegetables soup

Grilled shrimps with grilled vegetables

Diced fresh salad with dressing of choice

AFTERNOON SNACK

Strawberries

DINNER
Beef and vegetables soup

Grilled chicken with roast broccoli with cream cheese sauce

Fresh sliced salad

DAY 16

BREAKFAST

Baked egg with cream sauce, vegetables and sausages

Tea

MID MORNING SNACK
Sunflower seeds

LUNCH
Mutton and vegetables clear soup

Chicken and vegetables kebabs with cream cheese and mayo garlic sauce

Avocado and lettuce salad with lemon and olive oil dressing

AFTERNOON SNACK
Raspberry

DINNER
Chicken and broccoli cream soup

Grilled fish with lemon sauce

Diced green salad with sesame seed oil and vinegar dressing

DAY 17

BREAKFAST
Cheese omelet with green vegetables

Tea

MID MORNING SNACK
Mixed nuts

LUNCH
Clear vegetables and chicken soup

BBQ chicken with sautéed bell pepper and onion

Fresh cucumber and iceberg lettuce tossed with salad dressing

AFTERNOON SNACK
Strawberries

DINNER
Beef and vegetables clear soup

Baked chicken with mixed stir fried vegetables with cream cheese

Fresh sliced salad with lemon and olive oil dressing

DAY 18

BREAKFAST
Fried egg with roasted vegetables and cheese

Tea

MID MORNING SNACK
Mixed seeds

LUNCH
Clear beef and vegetables soup

Chicken roast with stir fried vegetables in peanut butter

Fresh diced salad with dressing of choice

AFTERNOON SNACK
Raspberries

DINNER
Clear beef and vegetables soup

Fried fish with coconut cream and lemon sauce

Avocado slices with cherry tomatoes

DAY 19

BREAKFAST
Soft boiled egg

Fried sausages with vegetables and cheese

Tea

MID MORNING SNACK
Mixed nuts

LUNCH
Clear vegetables and beef soup

Grilled mutton chops with roast mixed vegetables and lemon cheese sauce

Fresh sliced cucumber and lettuce salad

AFTERNOON SNACK
Strawberries

DINNER
Chicken and vegetables clear soup

Beef and green vegetables BBQ kebabs with stirfried vegetables

Fresh diced mixed salad with vinegar and olive oil dressing

DAY 20

BREAKFAST
Scrambled egg with cheese, vegetables and sausages

Tea

MID MORNING SNACK
Mixed seeds

LUNCH
Clear vegetables soup

Grilled beef with grilled vegetables

Fresh sliced salad with lemon and sesame seed oil

AFTERNOON SNACK
Raspberries

DINNER
Clear beef and vegetables soup

Fried fish with roast broccoli and cauliflower

Cherry tomato and cucumber salad

DAY 21

BREAKFAST
Cream cheese and vegetables omelet

Fried sausages

Tea

MID MORNING SNACK
Mixed nuts

LUNCH
Clear chicken and vegetables soup

Mutton and vegetables stew

Fresh avocado sliced

AFTERNOON SNACK
Strawberries

DINNER
Beef and vegetables clear soup

Roast beef with cream cheese and sautéed mixed vegetables

Sliced cucumber and lettuce

PHASE 2, FOURTH WEEK DIET PLAN

Add ½ a cup of unsweetened and unflavored yogurt in addition to what is allowed in the previous weeks

DAY 22

BREAKFAST
Scrambled eggs with cheese and vegetables

Fried sausages

Tea

MID MORNING SNACK
Mixed seeds

LUNCH
Cream of vegetables and chicken soup

Baked chicken with sautéed mixed vegetables

Fresh sliced avocado and olives with lemon juice

AFTERNOON SNACK
Strawberries

DINNER

Beef and vegetables cream soup

Beef steak with roast vegetables

Yogurt

DAY 23
BREAKFAST
Cheese omelet

Fried tofu with stir fried vegetables

Fried sausage

Tea

MID MORNING SNACK
Mixed nuts

LUNCH
Cream of mushroom, onion and chicken soup

Grilled chicken cutlet with saucy creamy grilled vegetables

Yogurt

AFTERNOON SNACK
Raspberries

DINNER
Beef and mixed vegetables cream soup

Beef and vegetables kebab

Fresh cucumber and lettuce diced

DAY 23
BREAKFAST
Fried egg with sautéed mixed vegetables

Grilled sausage

Tea

MID MORNING SNACK
Mixed seeds

LUNCH
Clear vegetables and beef soup

Roast chicken with roast vegetables

Yogurt

AFTERNOON SNACK
Strawberries

DINNER
Mutton and vegetables cream soup

Baked mutton with baked vegetables in cream cheese sauce

Cherry tomatoes and olives

DAY 24
BREAKFAST
Hard-boiled egg

Grilled mixed vegetables

Fried sausage with cream cheese

Tea

MID MORNING SNACK
Mixed nuts

LUNCH
Clear vegetables and beef soup

Fried minced meat balls with mixed grilled vegetables with peanut butter

Yogurt

AFTERNOON SNACK
Raspberries

DINNER
Beef and vegetables cream soup

Grilled fish with grilled vegetables

Fresh sliced salad

Day 25

BREAKFAST
Cheese omelet with vegetables

Fried sausage

Tea

MID MORNING SNACK
Mixed seeds

LUNCH
Clear vegetables and beef soup

Baked fish and vegetables with coconut cream and lemon sauce

Yogurt

AFTERNOON SNACK
Strawberries

DINNER
Clear vegetables and chicken soup
Beef BBQ kebab with grilled mixed vegetables

Sliced avocado

DAY 26

BREAKFAST
Scrambled egg with cheese, vegetables and tofu

Fried sausage

Tea

MID MORNING SNACK
Mixed nuts

LUNCH

Clear vegetables and mutton soup

Chicken steak with grilled vegetables and sour cream sauce

Yogurt

AFTERNOON SNACK

Raspberries

DINNER

Clear vegetables and beef soup

Fried mutton chops with roast vegetables

Cherry tomatoes and sliced cucumber

DAY 27

BREAKFAST

Baked egg with cheese, vegetables and tofu

Grilled sausage

Tea

MID MORNING SNACK

Mixed seeds

LUNCH

Clear vegetables and beef soup

Fried Chicken wings with grilled mixed vegetables

Yogurt

AFTERNOON SNACK

Strawberries

DINNER

Clear vegetables and mutton soup

Beef steak with roast vegetables

Sliced avocado

DAY 28

BREAKFAST

Omelet with cheese and vegetables

Grilled sausage

Tea

MID MORNING SNACK

Mixed nuts

LUNCH

Clear vegetables and chicken soup

Baked fish with grilled mixed vegetables

Yogurt

AFTERNOON SNACK

Raspberries

DINNER

Clear vegetables and beef soup

Beef steak with grilled vegetables

Lettuce diced

PHASE 2, FIFTH WEEK DIET PLAN

During the third week of phase 2 you can add one ounce of chickpeas or lentils in addition to your previous weekly plan

DAY 29

BREAKFAST

Scrambled egg

Fried sausage

Tea

MID MORNING SNACK

Mixed nuts

LUNCH

Lentils and vegetables soup
Baked chicken with roasted vegetables
Fresh salad

AFTERNOON SNACK
Strawberries with cream

DINNER
Clear chicken and vegetables soup
Fried fish with grilled vegetables
Yogurt

DAY 30
BREAKFAST
Cheese omelet
Fried tofu with vegetables
Tea

MID MORNING SNACK
Mixed seeds

LUNCH
Clear beef and vegetables soup
Grilled tuna with stir fried chickpeas
Fresh sliced salad

AFTERNOON SNACK
Raspberries with cream

DINNER
Clear beef broth
Chicken cutlet with stirfried vegetables
Yogurt

DAY 31

BREAKFAST
Soft boiled egg

Fried sausage

Avocado slices

Tea

MID MORNING SNACK
Mixed nuts

LUNCH
Lentil and vegetables soup

Grilled fish with stir fried vegetables

Fresh sliced salad with lemon juice and sesame seed oil

AFTERNOON SNACK
Strawberries with cream

DINNER
Clear chicken and vegetables soup

Chicken and vegetables kebab

Yogurt

DAY 32
BREAKFAST
Fried egg

Grilled sausage

Cherry tomatoes

Yogurt

Tea

MID MORNING SNACK
Mixed nuts

LUNCH

Clear soup

Baked chicken with baked vegetables

Chickpea, onion and tomato salad

AFTERNOON SNACK

Raspberries with cream

DINNER

Clear soup

Beef steak with grilled vegetables

Fresh sliced cucumber and lettuce

DAY 33
BREAKFAST

Hard-boiled egg

Fried sausage

Grilled broccoli

Tea

MID MORNING SNACK

Mixed nuts

LUNCH

Clear soup

Fried chicken drumsticks with roasted cauliflower and boiled chickpeas

Yogurt

AFTERNOON SNACK

Raspberries with cream

DINNER

Clear soup

Fried meat balls with grilled vegetables

Fresh sliced salad

DAY 34
BREAKFAST
Scrambled egg

Fried sausage

Avocado slices

Tea

MID MORNING SNACK
Mixed seeds

LUNCH
Clear soup

Grilled fish and whole lentils with cream cheese

Yogurt

AFTERNOON SNACK
Strawberries with cream

DINNER
Clear soup

Mutton baked chops with stirfried vegetables with garlic mayo sauce

Fresh diced salad

DAY 35
BREAKFAST
Cheese omelet

Grilled sausage

Roast vegetables

Tea

MID MORNING SNACK

Mixed seeds

LUNCH

Vegetables and lentils soup

Fried mutton chops with roasted vegetables

Yogurt

AFTERNOON SNACK

Raspberries with cream

DINNER

Clear soup

Baked fish with baked vegetables

Fresh diced salad

PHASE 2, SIXTH WEEK

During fourth week of phase 2, start adding 1 cup of tomato and vegetables juice, in addition to the previous diet plan.

DAY 36

BREAKFAST

Scrambled egg with vegetables

Strawberries with cream and nuts

Yogurt

Tea

MID MORNING SNACK

Tomato and vegetables juice

LUNCH

Chicken vegetables and lentils soup

Grilled chicken and stirfried broccoli with nutty cheese sauce

Fresh diced salad

AFTERNOON SNACK

Coconut water

DINNER

Clear broth

Fried fish with grilled cherry tomatoes

Avocado slices

DAY 37

BREAKFAST

Hard-boiled egg

Raspberries with cream and seeds

Yogurt

Tea

MID MORNING SNACK

Tomato and vegetables juice

LUNCH

Clear soup

Baked fish with grilled mixed vegetables

Fresh salad

AFTERNOON SNACK

Coconut water

DINNER

Clear soup

Fried meatballs with roast saucy vegetables

Sliced avocado

DAY 38

BREAKFAST
Cheese omelet

Strawberries with cream and nuts

Yogurt

Tea

MID MORNING SNACK
Tomatoes and vegetables soup

LUNCH
Clear soup

Grilled beef with stir fried vegetables

Avocado and olives slices

AFTERNOON SNACK
Coconut water

DINNER
Clear soup

Mutton roast with roast mixed vegetables

Sliced cucumber and lettuce with dressing of choice

DAY 39
BREAKFAST
Scrambled egg with cheese

Raspberries with cream and nuts

Yogurt

MID MORNING SNACK
Tomato and vegetables soup

LUNCH
Clear soup

Fried fish with mixed stir fried vegetables and lemon sauce

Cucumber slices

AFTERNOON SNACK

Coconut water

DINNER

Clear soup

Mutton and vegetables stew

Avocado slices

DAY 40

BREAKFAST

Fried egg with fried tofu

Strawberries with cream and nuts

Yogurt

Tea

MID MORNING SNACK

Tomato and vegetables juice

LUNCH

Clear soup

Baked chicken with grilled vegetables

Lettuce and cucumber slices

AFTERNOON SNACK

Coconut water

DINNER

Clear soup

Grilled fish with mixed roast vegetables

Avocado slices

DAY 41

BREAKFAST
Cheese omelet

Raspberries with cream and nuts

Yogurt

Tea

MID MORNING SNACK
Tomato and vegetables juice

LUNCH
Clear soup

Fried mutton chops

Vegetable puree with lemon and coconut sauce

Lettuce and olives, sliced

AFTERNOON SNACK
Coconut water

DINNER
Clear soup

Minced meatballs with sautéed green and red pepper

Avocado slices

DAY 42
BREAKFAST
Scrambled cheesy eggs with vegetables

Raspberries with cream and nuts

Yogurt

Tea

MID MORNING SNACK
Tomato and vegetables juice

LUNCH

Clear soup

Fried mutton chops

Mixed vegetables stew

Sliced cucumber and iceberg with lemon

AFTERNOON SNACK

Coconut water

DINNER

Clear soup

Chicken kebabs with garlic fried mixed vegetables and cheese

Avocado slices

CHAPTER 6. Safety and Effectiveness of Atkins Diet

The Atkins diet emphasizes utilization of fat stores of the body and energy from dietary fats and proteins, rather than depending on the carbohydrate sources of energy. When we switch from carbohydrates to fats and protein for energy, our body learns to adapt this change and tries to break down stores of body fats, in order to furnish energy.

There are three sources of energy-giving nutrients, proteins, fats and carbohydrates, which are also known as fuels for the body and macronutrients, as they form the bulk of our diet. Only in the absence of carbohydrates does the body system switch towards energy from fat. In the presence of carbohydrates, the body does not utilize the fat stores for energy efficiently; therefore, drastic cut down of carbohydrates is needed to break down adipose or fatty tissues of the body.

Sticking with Atkins diet may be challenging for a longer period of time. There have been quite a lot of studies to understand fully the effectiveness and risks attached with Atkins diet. Many have resulted in providing evidence for its effectiveness for reducing weight and improving blood cholesterol and triglycerides level. Atkins Nutritional Approach does not only deal in weight loss program, but claims to bring improvement in the lifelong eating habits. It is supposed to be beneficial for boosting energy, improving health problems, as well reducing overall body weight.

You may need to consult your physician before you start this diet if you are suffering from any kind of diseases or medical condition, especially diabetes, cardiovascular diseases or kidney related diseases and problems. The main focus of this diet is to create a balance of utilization between all the energy giving sources of food. This diet does not require you to trim your meat or avoid fats and oils, rather controlling of carbohydrates is the focal point.

Eating a high carbohydrate diet, which may include sugar, refined flour and carbohydrates rich sources of food products, is considered to be the real culprit behind many health conditions, problems, and diseases. The diet is still evolving and the older versions of this diet may slightly differ from the new ones. Exercise during the induction period is not advisable when the body is passing through a phase of changing dietary pattern and is struggling to achieve adjustment accordingly. It requires you to wait for at least two weeks before you start on any exercise regimen, in addition to your diet regimen.

There have been concerns by the health professionals for its overall safety, due to its high fat and high protein content. As we restrict dietary carbohydrates, we automatically switch toward high intake of fat and protein, as only these three energy giving nutrients constitute the bulk of our diet and therefore, are called macronutrients. This diet believes in keeping the follower fully satisfied while eating luxuriously. It begins from 20 grams net carbohydrates which keep on progressing to 5 grams each week till second phase and then 10 grams each week in the third phase.

In the initial period, the body uses up all the glucose stores in the body in the form of glycogen before going into ketosis. Fats, carbohydrates and proteins all three are energy giving nutrients and in the absence of one, the others will start furnishing energy. Excess of any will mainly be stored as body fat. When there are no supplies of glucose in the body to furnish energy, e. g. during starvation or fasting, the body learns to adapt and start utilizing other sources of energy. Fat catabolism and utilization produces ketone bodies, which become the primary source of energy, especially for brain function.

Our brain consumes around one fifth of our total energy consumption. Due to being mostly fat in its content, it needs many times more energy than any other body organ. Brains prefer glucose energy but only in the absence of glucose energy, will it learn to utilize the energy of ketones. Ketosis is not an abnormal state, but a normal condition happening during low consumption of carbohydrates.

Our body has to start burning fats when there are no carbohydrates in order to survive and to keep the body systems functioning. Utilization of fats encourages fat catabolism and break down of fatty muscles in the body and consequently, we lose weight. Atkins diet does not ask you to stop your carbohydrates forever, but only reduce it for a limited time period and then progressively it keeps on adding it. Surprising results of many research studies have shown that this diet is capable of reducing LDL (bad type) cholesterol while increasing HDL (good type) cholesterol.

There has been a concern of this diet being too high in protein, which may lead to progressive kidney diseases. The diet may also cause bad breath due to ketone bodies presence in the body. Due to ketosis, you may experience a number of side effects which may include nausea, fruity smell, and lack of appetite. Cost of the diet is one more consideration, as many people find high protein diet to be out of reach due to financial constraints.

Some people who have practiced this diet have experienced weight loss, which they say reappears after a short period of time. Lots of dietary planning is needed in this and many find it hard to accomplish the required results due to inadequate consistency. This diet is not advisable during pregnancy and lactation. There has been a lot of concern for its safety due to its high fat content, as well, because there has been correlation between a high fat diet and cardiovascular diseases.

Therefore, it may increase your chances of developing a heart related disease if you follow it for a longer period of time. In any case limiting the saturated fat is advisable in all conditions. Good fats and oils sources needed to be implemented during the active Atkins diet phases, especially if planning to adhere it for a longer period of time. From second phase and beyond, exercise in addition to diet may be helpful in reducing muscle loss happening and encourage muscle buildup.

Excess production of ketones may require the kidneys to function more to excrete these and therefore may over load the kidney function to remove toxicity. Constipation and diarrhea are some of the other complaints by people following this diet and may be due to lack of or overdose of fiber, respectively.

CHAPTER 7.   Recipes for Atkins Diet

BREAKFAST RECIPE
Baked egg with cauliflower
Ingredients

- Soy milk ½ cup
- Egg 1
- Cauliflower 1 cup, roasted in oven
- Cheddar cheese 1 ounce, grated
- Salt and pepper to taste
- Cilantro 1 tablespoon
- Olive oil ¼ cup

Method

- Mix egg and soy milk and cook in oil till dry.
- Mix all the ingredients together and spread on a baking dish and bake for ten minutes or till done in a pre-heated oven.
- Serve hot with unsweetened and decaffeinated tea of choice.

LUNCH RECIPE
Fried chicken with pureed vegetables and salad
Ingredients

- Mixed vegetables of choice, from allowed list, make puree 1 cup
- Lemon juice 1 tablespoon
- Garlic cloves 6 sliced
- Cream cheese 2 table spoons
- Sesame seed oil ¼ cup
- Salt and pepper to taste
- Chicken quarter 1, 4 to 5 ounces
- Ginger and garlic paste 1 tablespoon
- Mustard powder ¼ teaspoon
- Green chili paste 1 tablespoon
- Paprika ½ teaspoon
- Apple cider vinegar 1 tablespoon
- Olive oil for deep frying

Method

- Heat sesame seed oil and fry garlic slices till golden brown.
- Add pureed vegetables, cream cheese and lemon juice and mix well.
- Add salt and pepper to taste and mix well.
- Marinade chicken in rest of the ingredients except oil for some time.
- Deep fry chicken or bake it in a pre-heated oven till done.
- Serve hot chicken with pureed cooked vegetables mix and lettuce, avocado and cucumber slices.

DINNER
Grilled fish with stirfried vegetables and fresh salad
Ingredients

- Boneless fish fillet of choice 5 ounces
- Garlic paste 1 tablespoon
- Lemon juice 1 tablespoon
- Worcestershire sauce 1 tablespoon
- Salt and pepper to taste
- Mixed vegetables of choice from allowed list 1 cup diced
- Cumin seeds 1 teaspoon
- Oregano 1 tablespoon
- Sesame seed oil 4 tablespoons
- Salt and pepper to taste

Method

- Marinate fish fillet in garlic paste, lemon juice, Worcestershire sauce, salt and pepper for some time.
- Heat grill pan and grill fish on both sides until done.
- Fry cumin seeds in oil until brown.
- Add vegetables and rest of the ingredients and mix well.
- Stir fry for few minutes.
- Serve hot fish fillet with hot stirfried vegetables and fresh salad of choice.

CHAPTER 8. Frequently Asked Questions

Q1. What is Atkins diet for?

A1. Atkins diet is for weight reduction.

Q2. In addition to weight loss, what other health benefits does this diet offer?

A2. It may be helpful in reducing blood cholesterol level, insulin resistance and diabetes.

Q3. Can vegetarians follow this diet?

A3. Yes, vegetarians can exchange eggs, soy milk, tofu and tempeh for their meat and protein requirement.

Q4. For lifetime management, how much a carbohydrate is enough?

A4. Each person may have their own individual personal carbohydrate balance, which would not allow you to regain lost weight or cause carbohydrates cravings or hunger.

Q5. Can I have milk and milk products?

A5. You may have cheese and butter, but milk is not allowed during the induction phase as it contains lactose sugar.

Q6. Can I have artificial sweeteners?

A6. You may have Splenda, 1 to 3 packets per day.

Q7. What side effects are expected and how to avoid these?

A7. Constipation, dehydration, and leg cramps. Eat enough vegetables to avoid constipation, drink enough water and fluids to avoid dehydration and increase your electrolytes by adding salt and minerals in clear soup so that you may reverse any symptoms of water loss occurring during the induction period.

Q8. Can I have caffeine drinks?

A8. Try to limit your decaffeinated tea or coffee to two cups or 1 cup of regular or herbal tea.

CHAPTER 9. Conclusion

So, after in-depth learning and studying of this diet, we can conclusively say that this diet has a lot to offer, in regard to weight loss and therefore, could be opted in a systematic order. Persistence is a key to success and persistence is needed in this to achieve your overall target goal for weight loss.

Deviation from the dietary pattern may keep disrupting the whole body system and therefore, strict adherence to low carbohydrates dietary guidelines needs to be followed. A lot of variety is available in this and flexibility is allowed in the meal plan. Select from all the choices available and proceed accordingly.

Do not overindulge in food, but keep yourself self-satisfied at all times so that you do not start increasing your carbohydrates intake drastically. Have faith in yourself and learn the art of creative, quick cooking skills. Use the Atkins diet plan, follow it to suit your individual needs, and experience weight loss the Atkins way.

Made in the USA
Lexington, KY
17 September 2017